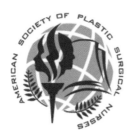

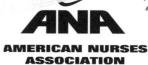

**AMERICAN NURSES
ASSOCIATION**

PLASTIC SURGERY NURSING:
SCOPE AND STANDARDS
OF PRACTICE

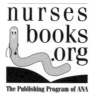

nurses
books
.org

The Publishing Program of ANA

AMERICAN NURSES ASSOCIATION
Silver Spring, MD
2005

Library of Congress Cataloging-in-Publication data

American Society of Plastic Surgical Nurses.
  Plastic surgery nursing : scope and standards of practice / American Society of Plastic Surgical Nurses.
    p. ; cm.
  Includes bibliographical references and index.
  ISBN-13: 978-1-55810-224-8
  1. Surgery, Plastic—Nursing—Practice—United States.   2. Surgery, Plastic—Nursing—Standards—United States.
  [DNLM: 1. Surgery, Plastic—nursing—United States.   2. Nursing—standards—United States.   3. Perioperative Nursing—United States. WY 161 P715 2005]   I. American Society of Plastic Surgical Nurses.   II. American Nurses Association.

  RD118.75.P56 2005
  617.9'50231—dc22   2005005263

The American Nurses Association (ANA) is a national professional association. This ANA publication—*Plastic Surgery Nursing: Scope and Standards of Practice*—reflects the thinking of the nursing profession on various issues and should be reviewed in conjunction with state board of nursing policies and practices. State law, rules, and regulations govern the practice of nursing, while *Plastic Surgery Nursing: Scope and Standards of Practice* guides nurses in the application of their professional skills and responsibilities.

Published by nursesbooks.org
The Publishing Program of ANA

American Nurses Association
8515 Georgia Avenue, Suite 400
Silver Spring, MD 20910
1-800-274-4ANA
http://www.nursingworld.org/

ANA is the only full-service professional organization representing the nation's 2.7 million Registered Nurses through its 54 constituent member associations. ANA advances the nursing profession by fostering high standards of nursing practice, promoting the economic and general welfare of nurses in the workplace, projecting a positive and realistic view of nursing, and lobbying the Congress and regulatory agencies on healthcare issues affecting nurses and the public.

The American Society of Plastic Surgical Nurses is committed to the enhancement of quality nursing care delivered to the patient undergoing plastic and reconstructive surgery. ASPSN promotes high standards of plastic and reconstructive surgical nursing practice and patient care through education, exchange of information, and scientific inquiry.

ISBN 978-1-55810-224-8   05SSPS   2M   04/05

First printing April 2005.

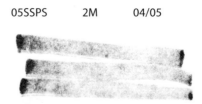

CONTENTS

Acknowledgments

Sharon Fritzsche, RN, MSN, APRN,BC
Judy Akin, RN, MSN, PHN

Special thanks to the Clinical Practice Committee Chairman Sharon D. Fritzsche MSN, RN, APRN,BC, and committee member Judy Akin, RN, MSN, PHN of the ASPSN for their invaluable insight and commitment to having the ASPSN be recognized as a specialty organization by the ANA. The ASPSN would also like to give thanks to Carol J. Bickford, PhD, RN, BC, Senior Policy Fellow, Department of Nursing Practice and Economics, for her guidance and reference in the development of the Scope of Practice Statement and revision of the Standards of Practice and Professional Performance for the ASPSN.

ANA Staff

Carol J. Bickford, PhD, RN,BC – Content Editor
Yvonne Humes, MSA
Winifred Carson, JD

Standards of Plastic Surgery Nursing Practice: Standards of Practice

Standard 1. Assessment
The plastic surgery nurse collects comprehensive data pertinent to the patient's health or the situation.

Standard 2. Diagnosis
The plastic surgery nurse analyzes the assessment data to determine the diagnosis or issues.

Standard 3. Outcomes Identification
The plastic surgery nurse identifies expected outcomes individualized to the patient or the situation.

Standard 4. Planning
The plastic surgery nurse develops a plan of care that prescribes strategies and alternatives to attain expected outcomes.

Standard 5. Implementation
The plastic surgery nurse implements the specified plan of care.

Standard 5a: Coordination of Care
The plastic surgery nurse coordinates care delivery.

Standard 5b: Health Teaching and Health Promotion
The plastic surgery nurse employs strategies to promote health and a safe environment.

Standard 5c: Consultation
The advanced practice registered nurse in plastic surgery provides consultation to influence the specified plan, enhance the abilities of others, and effect change.

Standard 5d: Prescriptive Authority and Treatment
The advanced practice nurse in plastic surgery uses prescriptive authority, procedures, referrals, treatments, and therapies in accordance with state and federal laws and regulations.

Standard 6. Evaluation
The plastic surgery nurse evaluates the patient's progress towards achievement of outcomes.

STANDARDS OF PLASTIC SURGERY NURSING PRACTICE: STANDARDS OF PRACTICE

STANDARD 7. QUALITY OF PRACTICE
The plastic surgery nurse systematically strengthens the quality and effectiveness of nursing practice.

STANDARD 8. EDUCATION
The plastic surgery nurse attains knowledge and competency that reflects current plastic surgery nursing practice.

STANDARD 9. PROFESSIONAL PRACTICE EVALUATION
The plastic surgery nurse evaluates their own nursing practice in relation to professional practice standards and guidelines, relevant statutes, rules, and regulations.

STANDARD 10. COLLEGIALITY
The plastic surgery nurse interacts with and contributes to the professional development of peers, colleagues, and other healthcare providers.

STANDARD 11. COLLABORATION
The plastic surgery nurse collaborates with patient, family, and others in the conduct of nursing practice.

STANDARD 12. ETHICS
The plastic surgery nurse integrates ethical provisions in all areas of practice.

STANDARD 13. RESEARCH
The plastic surgery nurse integrates research findings into practice.

STANDARD 14. RESOURCE UTILIZATION
The plastic surgery nurse considers factors related to safety, effectiveness, cost, and impact on practice in the planning and delivery of nursing services for the patient.

STANDARD 15. LEADERSHIP
The plastic surgery nurse provides leadership in the professional practice setting and the profession.

Scope of Plastic Surgery Nursing Practice

Definition of Plastic Surgery Nursing

Plastic surgery nursing specializes in the protection, maintenance, safety, and optimization of human bodily repair, restoration, and health before, during, and after plastic surgery procedures. This is accomplished through the nursing process, nursing diagnosis, and treatment of human response. Commitment to the nursing profession is reflected in service and advocacy for individuals, families, communities, and populations through to care, education, and ethics of plastic surgery issues and procedures.

Foundation of Plastic Surgery Nursing Practice

The specialty of plastic surgery has long pioneered surgical techniques and treatment strategies for human body and facial repair, reconstruction and replacement in cases of congenital diseases, traumatic injuries, and cancer reconstruction. Plastic surgery encompasses the skin, breast, trunk, craniomaxillofacial structures, musculoskeletal system, extremities, and external genitalia. Complex wounds, replantation, grafts, flaps, free tissue transfer, and use of implantable materials are also functions of plastic surgery surgical residencies. In addition, plastic surgery has extended surgical reconstruction to aid in the correction or enhancement of aesthetic surgical issues (American Board of Plastic Surgery 2003). Plastic surgery interventions encompass all ages, from the neonatal patient to the advanced geriatric patient. This requires specialized knowledge and treatment to ensure optimal patient outcomes. Plastic surgery is the only specialty recognized and supported by the American Board of Medical Specialties (ABMS 2000) that provides plastic, reconstructive, and aesthetic surgical procedures through board certification for plastic surgery.

Unfortunately, because of extensive media coverage of plastic surgery and increasing demands for aesthetic plastic surgery, procedures are being performed by other medical specialties without properly recognized or regulated board certifications or surgical residencies. The lack of regulation, specialized knowledge, and skill levels exposes individuals,

1

families, communities, and populations to unnecessary health and safety risks. Plastic surgery nurses are aware of the health risks associated with plastic surgery procedures. Plastic surgery nurses complement the plastic surgery specialty by a mutual focus on patient safety, health maintenance, and ultimate patient satisfaction and outcomes.

Plastic surgery nursing practice and standards reflect the nursing process, the nursing standards of both the American Nurses Association (ANA 1995, 2000, 2004), and the Association of periOperative Registered Nurses (AORN) standards of perioperative practice, and AORN standards of nursing practice (AORN 2001). Plastic surgery nursing requires specialized knowledge and skill levels for both the reconstructive and aesthetic aspects of surgical interventions during the consultation, preoperative, operative, and postoperative stages of the plastic surgery procedure process. Through the implementation and maintenance of specialized plastic surgery nursing standards of care and practice, individuals seeking or requiring plastic surgery intervention will be provided with education, knowledge, and care to ensure optimal surgical safety, protection, and outcomes.

Development of Plastic Surgery Nursing Practice

Plastic surgery nursing opportunities continue to expand as the demand for plastic surgery procedures and treatments grows, primarily in the United States. According to the American Society of Plastic Surgeons (ASPS 2004), over 15 million plastic surgery procedures and treatments were performed in 2003, compared to approximately 1.5 million in 1992. The need for awareness and knowledge of safety, ethical, and procedural issues will increase as plastic surgery becomes more common in a wide range of surgical environments.

As plastic surgery procedures increase, plastic surgery nursing will intersect with other specialties and bodies of knowledge. These specialties include, but are not limited to, neonatal, pediatrics, adults, geriatrics, general surgery, neurosurgery, advanced wound management, dermatology, burns, cancer, and trauma. Because of the physical and psychological complexities involved in caring for the plastic surgery patient, plastic surgery nursing integrates a holistic approach in the plan of care for the plastic surgery patient. Plastic surgery nursing skills and knowledge require a strong foundation in surgical principles, advanced wound care, bioethics, psychology, and critical thinking.

In response to the specialized needs of plastic surgery patients and the required nursing interventions, 100 surgical nurses convened in 1975 to establish the non-profit American Society of Plastic and Reconstructive Surgical Nurses (ASPRSN): the name was later changed to American Society of Plastic Surgical Nurses or ASPSN. These charter members sought to establish a specialized identity and share the knowledge needed to practice successfully. The mission and philosophy of the ASPSN were founded on principles of improving the quality of nursing care for the patient undergoing plastic or reconstructive surgery. The organization is committed to promoting high standards of nursing care and practice through shared knowledge, scientific inquiry, and continuing education, while supporting and encouraging collaborative interaction with clinical practice, administration, research, and academics (ASPSN 2002). The chronology of the development of plastic surgery nursing is summarized on page 4.

Today the ASPSN has over 1,700 active members working in various nursing environments: surgical facilities, home care, nursing research, outpatient care, hospitals, universities, private practice, and others. Members cover a wide range of educational levels, including associate degree, bachelor's degree, master's degree, advanced practice nurses, nurse first-assistants, and nurse educators. ASPSN serves its members through a national structure of four regions and a network of local chapters in the United States and Canada (ASPSN 2002). Through the development of unique plastic surgery knowledge, the plastic surgery nurse can properly respond to and communicate with a multidisciplinary team assigned to any plastic surgery patient.

As the field of plastic surgery evolves and incorporates other medical specialties, the climate for plastic surgery nursing requires continual review of related trends, products, and procedures. According to the current statistical data found on the ASPS and ASPSN web sites, new developments in plastic surgery include both surgical and non-surgical procedures and treatments. Between 1992 and 2002, tumor removal increased 35%, breast reconstruction 147%, scar revision 20%, and animal bite repair 35%. Aesthetic procedures showed an enormous increase between 1992 and 2002, with breast augmentation up 593%, breast lifts 575%, eyelid surgery 91%, facelifts 84%, forehead lifts 176%, buttock lifts 377%, and abdominoplasty 392%. Non-surgical treatments such as collagen injection increased by 139% in the same period. Some of the newest treatments increased dramatically in 2001 and 2002. These include Botox® injections—up 83%—and microdermabrasion—up 39% (ASPS 2004).

Development of Plastic Surgery Nursing

1975   The American Society of Plastic and Reconstructive Surgical Nurses (ASPRSN) holds its first national meeting in Toronto, Canada. Sherill Lee Schultz is the first president and founder.

1976   Thirteen local chapters of ASPRSN are established in the United States and Canada.

1980   ASPRSN creates the *Plastic Surgical Nursing Journal*.

1980   ASPRSN becomes the 22nd member of the National Federation for Specialty Nursing Organizations.

1984   The plastic surgical nursing bibliography is completed.

1989   The first edition of the *Core Curriculum for Plastic and Reconstructive Surgical Nursing* is published in1989 The Plastic Surgical Nursing Certification Board (PSNCB) is established.

1991   The first plastic surgical nursing certification examination (CPSN) is given.

1993   The National Institute of Nursing Research (NINR) is founded and helps move nursing research into the mainstream of research activities.

1995   ASPRSN establishes a Research Committee to assist ASPRSN nurses with research funds and priorities unique to plastic surgical nursing practice.

1996   The second edition of the *Core Curriculum for Plastic and Reconstructive Surgical Nursing* is published.

1998   ASPRSN creates a website: www.aspsn.org

2001   ASPRSN simplifies its name to the American Society of Plastic Surgical Nurses (ASPSN).

2004   Recognition of the specialty and drafting of the ASPSN–ANA specialty standards, *Surgical Nursing: Scope and Standards of Practice*

Plastic surgery nurses help to regulate quality of care before, during, and after plastic surgical procedures and treatments to ensure proper health maintenance, safety, and restoration. Plastic surgery nurses determine the specific nursing intervention needed for each individual undergoing a plastic surgical procedure or treatment, in accordance with the nursing process (assessment, diagnosis, outcome identification, planning, implementation, and evaluation). This nursing specialty continues to develop the knowledge base for evidence-based practice through research into plastic surgery procedures, treatments, and issues.

One goal of plastic surgery nursing is to secure the foundation for safety. This is accomplished through stronger regulations, increased education, and awareness among patients, families, communities, and populations seeking or requiring plastic surgery-related interventions.

Educational Preparation and Requirements for Plastic Surgery Nursing

Plastic surgery nursing training embodies *Nursing's Social Policy Statement* (ANA 2003) from novice to expert nursing practice. Advanced education and nursing practice in plastic surgery build on generic practice. Education, experience, and increased familiarity with plastic surgery procedures and outcomes will increase knowledge and skill levels needed to care for the plastic surgery patient.

Due to the complexities of plastic surgery, including psychological and psychosocial factors, plastic surgery nurses require a minimum of two years of basic surgical nursing experience before starting graduate courses or certification in plastic surgery nursing. During the two years of basic surgical nursing, student nurses learn plastic surgery fundamentals from ASPSN introduction courses, core curriculum materials, and seminars pertaining to plastic surgery education, procedures, and issues.

The list on page 6 provides an overview of the minimum requirements for plastic surgery nursing.

Roles of Plastic Surgery Nurses

The roles of the plastic surgery nurse derive from the professional development of specific standards of care, required educational guidelines, and practice environments and settings for the plastic surgery patient.

Media coverage has deluged our society with information about plastic surgery that is often questionable, confusing the general public about its seriousness and providing economic incentives for physicians. Both the increasing awareness in our society (accurate and otherwise) of plastic surgery and the ambiguities of cosmetic surgery call for more nursing, consumer, and patient education interventions by plastic surgery nurses to help clarify misconceptions.

Minimum Requirements for Plastic Surgery Nursing

- Licensure as a registered nurse (RN) within the designated state of practice
- Education:
  - Minimum requirement—Associate degree from an accredited college of nursing
  - Preferred—Bachelor of Science degree in nursing from an accredited college of nursing
- Advanced knowledge in surgical principles, anatomy, and physiology for a specified age group (neonate, child, adolescent, adult, geriatric)
- Advanced knowledge in one or more of the following:
  - Wound care, burns, trauma, cancer-related disfigurements
  - Scar management, body image, health assessment, nutrition
- Continuing education and knowledge of current plastic surgery trends, issues, and procedures
- Certification—Registered nurses can earn specialty certification in plastic surgery nursing by meeting eligiblity requirements and passing the CPSN exam. A registered nurse must have two or more years experience working in plastic surgery nursing to become eligible to take the CPSN exam. The CPSN exam is a method to test and validate the skills, knowledge, and ability of the plastic surgery nurse. The Plastic Surgical Nursing Certification Board, comprised of registered nurses with content expertise in plastic surgery nursing, has oversight of the CPSN exam and collaborates and participates with other specialty nursing certifying bodies through the National Specialty Nursing Certifying Organization (NSNCO) in addressing issues related to certification, licensure, education, and research. Certification is suggested but not required.

One of the goals of plastic surgery nursing is to reach and educate other nurses and nursing students about plastic surgery issues, procedures, and current trends. Communication and interaction with other nursing specialties about the role of plastic surgery nurses will provide a broader understanding and knowledge base for nursing collaboration. Plastic surgery nurses help build the foundations of knowledge and education for improved outcomes, safety, health maintenance, and health awareness. It is through education and research that the practice of plastic surgery nursing can be recognized as a specialty.

General Nursing Role

Associate or bachelor degree nurses beginning clinical practice in their first year of licensure are encouraged to gain knowledge and develop skill levels associated with basic surgical principles in preparation for later specialization in plastic surgery nursing. Registered nurses who enter the field of plastic surgery must have a well-rounded knowledge base about various patient populations. The scope of knowledge required for the plastic surgery nurse varies with the area of practice interest, previous nursing experience, and level of educational preparation. The general level plastic surgery nurse will progress into a more expert role with experience, training, and additional education, which may include preparation for plastic surgery nursing subspecialties such as neonatal, pediatrics, general surgery, neurosurgery, advanced wound management, dermatology, burns, cancer, trauma, and operating room environments.

Advanced Practice Role

Advanced practice plastic surgery nursing roles are increasing in reaction to personal, professional, and societal needs. Nurse practitioner (NP) and clinical nurse specialist (CNS) are two of the roles included under the role of *advanced practice nurse (APN)* or *advanced practice registered nurse (APRN)*. The advanced practice plastic surgery nurse is a registered nurse with a master's or higher degree in nursing. Credentialing is available for the CNS or NP advanced practice nurse in the specialty of plastic surgery.

Advanced practice registered nurses play a significant role in meeting the needs of the plastic surgery patient. Advanced practice nurses in plastic surgery are valuable to a practice because of their ability to use independent judgment in clinical decision-making, and to provide skilled, quality, and detailed advanced nursing care across the continuum. An advanced practice nurse in plastic surgery has the knowledge and training to provide comprehensive health assessments, differential diagnoses, and treatments for plastic surgery patients and others. Advanced practice nurses in plastic surgery advocate health maintenance, health promotion, and wellness.

Advanced practice nurses in plastic surgery serve as resources and consultants to other healthcare disciplines. The advanced practice nurse is instrumental in facilitating and conducting research in plastic surgery. The advanced practice nurse also plays a key role in providing continuity of care for the plastic surgery patient. Legislation has now made prescriptive authority and third-party reimbursement possible for the advanced practice nurse in the plastic surgery arena. The roles of the advanced practice nurse in plastic surgery are developing and expanding. National certification in advanced practice plastic surgery nursing is recommended. Many advanced practice nurses in plastic surgery have advanced practice certifications in other areas.

Educator Role

As the need for plastic surgery education becomes more evident, so is the need to disseminate education throughout the nursing field and the general population. Nurse educators promote educational clarity, standards, knowledge, and safety related to plastic surgery procedures, issues, and outcomes. In this document, the plastic surgery nurse in an educator role will be referred to as the *plastic surgery nurse educator*.

A plastic surgery nurse educator is educated at the bachelor, graduate, or doctorate degree level with a focus on plastic surgery education. Plastic surgery nurse educators also comply with and support state educational requirements to teach at community or university institutions according to their educational background. At the graduate or doctoral level, the plastic surgery nurse educator has the opportunity to facilitate and develop focused education, curriculums, and research in plastic surgery.

A plastic surgery nurse educator develops instruction, guidelines, materials, and programs for nurses during nursing school rotations, distant learning experiences, and in various practices, environments, and settings related to plastic surgery. A plastic surgery nurse educator also provides education for local and national communities on plastic surgery and relevant resources.

A plastic surgery nurse educator conducts a needs assessment to help establish educational requirements in various practice environments and settings. A plastic surgery nurse educator functions as an educator and a liaison between the plastic surgeon or advanced practice plastic surgery nurse and the patient to help ensure continuity of care, health promotion, and health maintenance. Providing educational materials during the consultation, preoperative, and postoperative stages is key to educational consistency among staff members, plastic surgeons, advanced practice plastic surgery nurses, and plastic surgery patients. A plastic surgery nurse educator provides an appropriate climate for learning, and ensures that the learners are actively involved in the learning process and in identification of learning outcomes through in-service updates on current issues, procedures, or products related to plastic surgery. Plastic surgery nurse educators evaluate the effectiveness and outcomes of various educational strategies and then provide a revised plan to correct any shortcomings.

A plastic surgery nurse educator is a member of a multidisciplinary team, and functions as a consultant, change agent, leader, and resource to other nursing and healthcare disciplines. Plastic surgery nurse educators help to conduct research and disseminate findings. A plastic surgery nurse educator requires a strong knowledge base of teaching and learning theories, curriculum development, research, test and measurement evaluation methods, critical thinking skills, and quality improvement techniques.

Plastic Surgery Nursing Research

Research is a group of activities designed to expand knowledge. Research includes utilization of theories, principles, or relationships. Research helps to streamline or reorganize existing bodies of information, to verify existing theory, and to apply existing knowledge.

Both reconstructive and aesthetic surgical outcomes need to be evaluated and assessed for improved patient outcomes and health management. In order to introduce new materials, refine educational guidelines, and provide valid evidence to support or discard current practice regimens, nursing research is crucial. Nurses must demonstrate scientifically that nursing interventions make a positive difference in the outcomes and health status of plastic surgery patients. Nurses need research-based knowledge to improve decision-making skills regarding proper care for plastic surgery patients and to implement and evaluate care management. Because of the psychological and clinical aspects of plastic surgery, both the qualitative and quantitative approaches to research can be used to evaluate plastic surgery research criteria and outcomes.

Through the translation and dissemination of research, nursing will continue as an independent professional entity in health care, fulfilling its responsibility in collegial relationships with other professionals. Application of research findings in practice is important to improve patient outcomes and quality of life, enhance nursing practice, and deliver effective, quality health care. The current research of nursing professionals is building a solid theoretical foundation for the plastic surgery nursing practice of the future. Topics of plastic surgery nursing research include nursing strategies different from the activities and actions of other disciplines, outcome measures, program evaluation, nursing interventions, and historical issues of ethics and policy. Knowledge of plastic surgery nursing research is needed to enhance the professional practice of all nurses, including both consumers of research (those who read, evaluate, and implement practice-based changes from studies) and producers (those who undertake research studies).

Practice Environments and Settings for the Plastic Surgery Nurse

The plastic surgery nurse provides care for patients and their families or caretakers in a variety of settings and locations that include hospitals, outpatient ambulatory surgery centers, office-based surgery centers, and private practice. The plastic surgery nurse is prepared to educate and provide comprehensive care to patients in a safe and regulated environment. The plastic surgery nurse provides competent, ethical, and appropriate nursing care to help improve surgical experiences and outcomes. In order to determine and implement the plan of care, and to ensure optimal outcomes for the plastic surgery patient, the plastic surgery nurse encourages and facilitates consultations, communication, and collaboration with other healthcare team members.

Plastic surgery nurses are also knowledgeable of proper policies, procedures, contracts, and regulations, including those for compliance with the Health Insurance Portability and Accountability Act (HIPAA), in appropriate and designated plastic surgery settings. Plastic surgery nurses know and comply with the requirements for federal, state, local, insurance, and accreditation agency standards. Plastic surgery nurses help promote safer surgical services for the plastic surgery patient.

Hospital

The plastic surgery nurse working in the hospital environment may care for plastic surgery patients in a variety of specialty departments or units. These include, among others, emergency departments, operating rooms, surgical floor/units, burn units, critical care units, neonatal units, pediatrics, and oncology. Plastic surgery nursing within the hospital environment is multidimensional and includes skills, functions, roles, and responsibilities that evolve from the body of knowledge specific to plastic surgery nursing. These dimensions are apparent in the plastic surgery nursing roles, processes, and characteristics. The plastic surgery nurse practicing in the hospital environment may provide assessment, analysis, nursing diagnosis, planning, implementation of interventions, outcome identification, and evaluation of patients in all age groups whose care requires plastic surgery interventions, procedures, and/or treatments. Regulatory factors pertinent to plastic surgery nurses working in the hospital environment include the Joint Commission on Accreditation of Healthcare Organizations (JCAHO); specific hospital rules and regulations; and rules, regulations, and guidelines governed by each state board of nursing that ensure public safety.

Outpatient /Ambulatory Surgery Center

The plastic surgery nurse working in the outpatient/ambulatory surgery center demonstrates the appropriate skills, knowledge, competencies, and abilities to provide proper and safe nursing care for the plastic surgery patient in the preoperative, operative, and postoperative stages of the plastic surgery procedure. The outpatient/ambulatory surgery center must be accredited or certified by the appropriate surgery center accreditation for the state where the plastic surgery nurse holds a license.

The plastic surgery nurse functions within the guidelines of the Accreditation Association for Ambulatory Health Care (AAAHC), the AAAHC Institute for Quality Improvement (IQI), and the American Association for Accreditation of Ambulatory Surgery Facilities (AAAASF). The plastic surgery nurse promotes higher quality surgical outcomes by maintaining standards, measuring performance, and providing consultation and education. The plastic surgery nurse complies with and promotes the laws and regulations governing the operation of the facility, such as Occupational Safety and Health Administration (OSHA) standards for bloodborne pathogens and hazardous waste; the Americans with Disabilities Act; and appropriate federal, state, and local laws. The plastic surgery nurse working in an outpatient/ambulatory surgery center maintains the plastic surgery nursing standards of practice and standards of professional performance.

Office-Based Surgery Center

According to ASPS (2004) statistical data, 56% of aesthetic plastic surgery procedures and 51% of reconstructive plastic surgery procedures are performed in a plastic surgeon's office. This poses risks if the office does not have a properly accredited or regulated surgery facility. Public awareness and understanding of proper accreditation and regulation are needed to provide clarity and guidance when considering plastic surgery. The plastic surgery nurse is aware of the potential confusion surrounding office-based surgery and can be instrumental in providing proper education about accreditation and regulation for other nurses, patients, and communities. The plastic surgery nurse working in an office-based surgery center demonstrates the appropriate skills, knowledge, competencies, and abilities to provide proper nursing care for the plastic surgery patient.

The plastic surgery nurse's role in the office-based surgery center includes the consultation, preoperative, postoperative, and follow-up stages of the plastic surgery procedure. Assessment, education, planning and intervention are part of the plastic surgery nurse's role during each stage of a plastic surgery procedure. The plastic surgery nurse helps to improve the quality of care by maintaining standards, including the Standards of Plastic Surgery Nursing, measuring performance, and providing education within the specific office-based surgery center.

The plastic surgery nurse working in the office-based surgery center complies with, and promotes compliance with, the laws and regulations governing the operation of the office-based surgery facility, such as the OSHA standards for bloodborne pathogens and hazardous waste; the

Americans with Disabilities Act; and appropriate federal, state, and local laws. The plastic surgery nurse should also know and address compliance with the guidelines of the Accreditation Association for Ambulatory Health Care (AAAHC), the AAAHC Institute for Quality Improvement (IQI) and the American Association for Accreditation of Ambulatory Surgery Facilities, Inc. (AAAASF).

Private Practice

The private practice setting provides plastic surgery nurses with the opportunity to interact directly with the patient throughout the plastic surgery process and recovery. Mutual goals and surgical expectations are assessed on a more personal and interactive level than other settings. Preoperative and postoperative evaluations are more accessible and can provide valuable information when evaluating quality of outcomes. The plastic surgery nurse in private practice is encouraged to have two or more years of plastic surgery nurse experience within a hospital or outpatient/ambulatory surgery center. The plastic surgery nurse in private practice requires competence and confidence to respond appropriately and safely to plastic surgery patients and their needs.

The plastic surgery nurse working in a physician-owned and -supervised private practice may possess an associate degree or higher, and function quite like an advanced practice nurse or nurse educator in the practice environment. Responsibilities may include assessment of an individual patient's needs, educational material development, assisting physicians or advanced practice plastic surgery nurses, staff education, and in-service and patient education. The plastic surgery nurse assesses educational needs and then provides educational material and instruction on the plastic surgery procedure.

The plastic surgery nurse also provides preoperative and postoperative counseling regarding technical aspects of the surgical procedure, documented health assessment, pertinent mutual goal planning, and psychosocial assessment and support. The plastic surgery nurse may provide consumer education about selecting an appropriate plastic surgery facility and provider that will meet the patient's needs and provide the best outcomes. The plastic surgery nurse in private practice provides follow-up communication and evaluation to ensure quality of care, health maintenance, and proper documentation for the plastic surgery patient. The plastic surgery nurse in private practice maintains the plastic surgery nursing standards of practice and standards of professional performance.

Patient Population

The plastic surgery nurse interacts with and cares for patients who require or desire plastic or reconstructive surgery for enhancement or restoration purposes. The plastic surgery nurse also interacts with and educates families of plastic surgery patients, as well as communities, regarding plastic surgery procedures and issues. The plastic surgery nurse has the special knowledge and skills needed to meet the needs of the patient population. The plastic surgery nurse provides care for patients in a variety of settings, age groups, and populations, including neonatal, pediatric, adult, geriatric, general surgery, neurosurgery, advanced wound management, dermatology, burns, cancer, and trauma patients.

Patients receiving care and education from a plastic surgery nurse require a thorough understanding of procedures, personal expectations, and mutual goal setting in order to achieve maximum satisfaction and health maintenance. Plastic surgery nurses help patients to deal with perceived or altered body image, perceived surgical outcomes, fears, and learning needs associated with a surgical intervention. Patients undergoing plastic surgery may encounter psychological, emotional, and physical imbalances during the recovery phase. Managing the psychological discord associated with physical alterations requires specialized knowledge and education.

Reconstructive Plastic Surgery Patient Population

Reconstructive plastic surgery includes skin, breast, trunk, craniomaxillofacial structures, musculoskeletal system, extremities, and external genitalia. Nurses in reconstructive plastic surgery require specialized knowledge related to complex wounds, replantation, grafts, flaps, free tissue transfer, and use of implantable materials reconstruction or repair due to cancer, trauma, burns, superficial injury, congenital defects, or disease. Plastic surgery nurses help the patient to express psychological, physical, and psychosocial needs in order to regain or rediscover coping strategies and successful interaction with society. Thorough assessment and documentation before, during, and after surgery is essential for proper evaluation of patient outcomes.

Aesthetic Plastic Surgery Patient Population

Aesthetic plastic surgery includes skin, breast, trunk, craniomaxillofacial structures, musculoskeletal system, extremities, and external genitalia. Aesthetic plastic surgery may be performed after reconstructive surgery to improve overall results. Plastic surgery nurses require specialized knowledge associated with reconstructive surgical principles to assist in the successful recovery and outcomes of the aesthetic surgery patient. Aesthetic surgery includes adjustment, enhancement, and alteration according to each patient's request for plastic surgery intervention. Thorough assessment and documentation before, during, and after surgery is essential for proper evaluation of patient outcomes.

Ethics and Advocacy in Plastic Surgery Nursing

Ethics is a fundamental part of nursing. Ethical awareness, judgments, and decisions are founded on a combination of principles, theories, and moral foundations. Nursing ethics are based on care and the actions of caring, to enhance and protect patient well-being. Plastic surgery nurses are expected to comply with and promote the ethical ideals, model, code, and principles of the nursing profession. *Code of Ethics for Nurses with Interpretive Statements* (ANA 2001) is the framework on which plastic surgery nurses base ethical analysis and decision-making, and on which standards are based. The plastic surgery nurse is also an advocate for the patient and provides care in a non-discriminatory and non-judgmental way. Patient advocacy means preservation of patient autonomy, execution of clinical judgments, and management of ethical issues.

The plastic surgery nurse maintains the plastic surgery standards of practice and standards of professional performance in each type of practice environment to help ensure the safety, quality of care, and the highest level of health maintenance or health restoration for the plastic surgery patient. The plastic surgery nurse promotes an ethical practice environment by serving as a patient advocate. The plastic surgery nurse's attitude and performance reflect compassion and understanding of a patient's self-respect, cultural beliefs, sovereignty, and rights to self-determination and privacy. Plastic surgery nurses implement the principles of autonomy, nonmaleficence, beneficence, and justice when interacting with patients requiring or desiring plastic surgery intervention. Plastic surgery nurses are aware of the many ethical considerations associated with plastic surgery. These include misleading advertising, the aging population, insurance reimbursement, and other matters. Public awareness of these issues is key to proper acknowledgment of the physical and emotional health risks of plastic surgery.

Misleading Advertising

Advertisements for plastic surgery are found on the Internet, television, magazines, and radio. Many plastic or cosmetic surgery advertisements do not disclose risks, recovery time, contraindications, physician credentials, type of board certification, or type of surgical facility. Plastic surgery nurses encourage consumers interested in plastic surgery to inquire about the physician, the surgical environment, and the procedure in detail in order make an informed decision. The ABPS (2003) does not approve of plastic surgery advertising that raises unrealistic, false, or misleading expectations. Public awareness of advertising statements that minimize risks is one goal of plastic surgery nursing in its community education campaigns.

The Aging Population

The quest for a more youthful appearance to complement longevity is spreading among the aging population in our society. Aging adults are considered vulnerable because of age-related physical and cognitive changes that make them more susceptible to health risks during and after surgery. According to the ASPS statistical chart for age distribution (2004), aesthetic plastic surgery procedures for ages 65 and over increased 5 from 2002 to 2003. Over 400,000 aesthetic plastic surgery procedures were performed on patients 65 and older in 2003. Plastic surgery nurses must be aware of the specialized needs of the aging population, as well as the ethical considerations associated with aesthetic surgery requests by patients. Opportunities for plastic surgery nurses to serve as patient advocates for the aging population are increasing as the demand for aesthetic surgery procedures and treatments increases.

Insurance Reimbursements

The ethics of insurance reimbursements for plastic surgery procedures is still controversial. The question centers around how insurance companies view reconstructive vs. aesthetic surgery. Reconstructive plastic surgery may be needed as a result of cancer, trauma, burns, superficial injury, congenital defects, or disease. Aesthetic plastic surgery may then follow reconstructive plastic surgery in order to improve results. Insurance reimbursements may not be granted for those requiring multiple surgeries for the best possible outcomes. A plastic surgery nurse in a plastic surgery practice environment may act as a patient advocate or a change agent to help improve insurance reimbursements.

STANDARDS OF PLASTIC SURGERY NURSING PRACTICE
STANDARDS OF PRACTICE

All plastic surgery nursing practice standards and documentation will abide by current statutes, rules, regulations, and the guidelines of the Health Insurance Portability and Accountability Act (HIPAA).

STANDARD 1. ASSESSMENT
The plastic surgery nurse collects comprehensive data pertinent to the patient's health or the situation.

Measurement Criteria:

The plastic surgery nurse:

- Collects data in a systematic and ongoing process.

- Includes the patient, family, significant others, and appropriate healthcare providers in the holistic data collection process.

- Records pertinent data in the patient's permanent medical record,

- Is sensitive to cultural diversity, ethnicity, gender, and lifestyle choices.

- Prioritizes data collection according to the patient's immediate health condition, or the anticipated needs of the plastic surgery patient or situation.

- Uses appropriate evidence-based assessment techniques and instruments in collecting pertinent data.

- Uses analytical models and problem-solving tools.

- Synthesizes available data, information, and knowledge relevant to the situation to identify patterns and variances.

- Documents relevant data in a retrievable format.

Additional Measurement Criteria for the Advanced Practice Registered Nurse:

The advanced practice registered nurse in plastic surgery:

- Conducts in-depth and comprehensive assessments based on a synthesis of individual and family health.

Continued ▶

- Bases assessments on advanced knowledge in the field of plastic surgery.

- Initiates and interprets diagnostic tests and procedures relevant to the current status of plastic surgery patient.

STANDARD 2. DIAGNOSIS

The plastic surgery nurse analyzes the assessment data to determine the diagnosis or issues.

Measurement Criteria:

The plastic surgery nurse:

- Derives the diagnosis and issues from the assessment data obtained during interview, physical examination, diagnostic test, or diagnostic procedures.

- Bases the diagnosis on actual or potential responses to alterations in health.

- Discusses and validates the diagnoses or issues with the plastic surgery patient, significant others, and other appropriate healthcare providers when possible.

- Documents the diagnosis or issues, and communicates them in a manner that facilitates the plan of care, interventions, expected outcomes, and plan for the plastic surgery patient.

Additional Measurement Criteria for the Advanced Practice Registered Nurse:

The advanced practice registered nurse in plastic surgery:

- Systematically compares and contrasts clinical findings of the plastic surgery patient with normal and abnormal variations and developmental events when formulating a differential diagnosis.

- Utilizes complex data and information obtained during interview, examination, and diagnostic procedures, and initiates further appropriate diagnostic tests to complete the diagnostic analysis.

- Assists staff in building and sustaining competency in the diagnostic process.

STANDARD 3. OUTCOMES IDENTIFICATION

The plastic surgery nurse identifies expected outcomes individualized to the patient or the situation.

Measurement Criteria:

The plastic surgery nurse:

- Jointly formulates expected plastic surgery patient outcomes with input from the plastic surgery patient, family, significant others, and healthcare providers when possible and appropriate.

- Derives culturally appropriate expected outcomes from the diagnoses.

- Considers available resources, associated risks, benefits, costs, current scientific evidence, and clinical expertise when developing expected outcomes of the plastic surgery patient.

- Determines expected outcomes with reflection and sensitivity to the plastic surgery patient, the patient's values, ethical considerations, environment or situation, cultural diversity, ethnicity, gender, and lifestyle choices.

- Determines expected outcomes with consideration of associated risks, benefits, costs, and current scientific evidence.

- Includes a time estimate for attainment of expected outcomes.

- Develops expected outcomes that realistically consider the plastic surgery patient's current and potential physical capabilities and provide direction for continuity of care.

- Modifies expected outcomes based on changes in the status of the plastic surgery patient or evaluation of the situation.

- Documents expected outcomes as measurable goals.

Additional Measurement Criteria for the Advanced Practice Registered Nurse:

The advanced practice registered nurse in plastic surgery:

- Identifies expected outcomes that include scientific evidence and are attainable through implementation of evidence-based practices.

- Identifies expected outcomes that incorporate cost and clinical effectiveness, patient satisfaction, and continuity and consistency among providers.

- Supports the use of clinical guidelines associated with positive plastic surgery patient outcomes.

- Modifies expected outcomes based on changes in the plastic surgery patient's or family's health status.

STANDARD 4. PLANNING

The plastic surgery nurse develops a plan of care that prescribes strategies and alternatives to attain expected outcomes.

Measurement Criteria:

The plastic surgery nurse:

- Individualizes the plan of care to the physical, emotional, psychosocial, cultural, and spiritual needs, desires, and resources of the plastic surgery patient and family.

- Develops the plan of care in collaboration with the plastic surgery patient, family, and other healthcare providers as appropriate.

- Documents strategies in the plan appropriate to each of the identified diagnoses or issues, and that may include strategies for health promotion, disease prevention, and restoration of health for the plastic surgery patient.

- Provides for continuity of care in the plan.

- Integrates an implementation pathway or timeline within the plan.

- Institutes the plan priorities with the plastic surgery patient, family, and others as appropriate.

- Uses the plan to guide treatment of the plastic surgery patient by other members of the healthcare team.

- Defines the plan that reflects current state laws, policies, regulations, and standards.

- Integrates current trends and scientific research in the planning process.

- Considers the economic impact of the plan on the plastic surgery patient.

- Utilizes standardized language or recognized terminology to record the plan.

Additional Measurement Criteria for the Advanced Practice Registered Nurse:

The advanced practice registered nurse in plastic surgery:

- Identifies assessment, diagnostic strategies, and therapeutic interventions in the plan that reflect current evidence, including data, research, literature, and expert clinical knowledge.

- Selects or designs strategies to meet the multifaceted needs of complex plastic surgery patients.

- Includes the synthesis of the plastic surgery patient's values and beliefs regarding nursing and medical therapies within the plan.

STANDARD 5. IMPLEMENTATION

The plastic surgery nurse implements the identified plan of care.

Measurement Criteria:

The plastic surgery nurse:

- Implements the plan of care for the plastic surgery patient in a safe and timely manner.

- Documents implementation of the plan, including any changes to or omissions from the plan.

- Employs evidence-based interventions and treatments for the plastic surgery patient that are relevant to the diagnosis or problem.

- Selects and implements interventions based on available community resources and systems.

- Collaborates with other appropriate members of the interdisciplinary healthcare team to implement the plan of care for the plastic surgery patient.

Additional Measurement Criteria for the Advanced Practice Registered Nurse:

The advanced practice registered nurse in plastic surgery:

- Facilitates in the utilization of systems and community resources to implement the plan of care for the plastic surgery patient.

- Supports the collaboration with other appropriate members of the interdisciplinary healthcare team to implement the plan of care for the plastic surgery patient.

- Incorporates new information, data, and strategies to initiate change in nursing care practices if preferred outcomes are not achieved.

STANDARD 5A: COORDINATION OF CARE

The plastic surgery nurse coordinates care delivery.

Measurement Criteria:

The plastic surgery nurse:

- Coordinates implementation of the plan of care.
- Documents the coordination of the care and treatments.

Additional Measurement Criteria for the Advanced Practice Registered Nurse:

The advanced practice registered nurse in plastic surgery:

- Provides leadership in the coordination of multidisciplinary health care for integrated delivery of patient care services.
- Synthesizes data and information to recommend necessary system and community support measures, including any environmental adjustments.
- Coordinates system and community resources that enhance delivery of care across continuums.
- Considers the plastic surgery patient's and family's complex needs and desired outcomes when coordinating and negotiating health-related and other specialized care needs.

Standard 5b: Health Teaching and Health Promotion

The plastic surgery nurse employs strategies to promote health and a safe environment.

Measurement Criteria:

The plastic surgery nurse:

- Provides education in such topics as healthy lifestyles, risk-reducing behaviors, developmental needs, activities of daily living, and preventive self-care.

- Promotes quality of life for the plastic surgery patient and family members by maximizing, restoring, and maintaining functional status to promote activities of daily living, as appropriate to the plastic surgery patient and the improvement of their safety and welfare.

- Utilizes health promotion and health teaching methods appropriate to the situation, and that recognize developmental level, culture, learning needs, readiness and ability to learn, language preference, and other factors of the plastic surgery patient and the family.

- Seeks opportunities for feedback and evaluation of the effectiveness of the strategies and interventions used.

Additional Measurement Criteria for the Advanced Practice Registered Nurse:

The advanced practice registered nurse in plastic surgery:

- Synthesizes empirical evidence on risk behaviors, learning theories, behavioral change theories, motivational theories, epidemiology, and other related theories and frameworks when designing health information and patient education.

- Designs health information and patient education appropriate to the plastic surgery patient's developmental level, learning needs, health, cultural beliefs and practices, and readiness to learn.

- Evaluates health information resources, such as the Internet and peer-reviewed journals, within the area of plastic surgery for accuracy, readability, and comprehensibility to help plastic surgery patients access quality health information.

STANDARD 5C: CONSULTATION

The advanced practice registered nurse in plastic surgery provides consultation to influence the specified plan, enhance the abilities of others, and effect change.

Measurement Criteria for the Advanced Practice Registered Nurse:

The advanced practice registered nurse in plastic surgery:

- Synthesizes clinical data, theoretical frameworks, and evidence when providing consultation.

- Facilitates the effectiveness of a consultation by involving the plastic surgery patient and other stakeholders in the decision-making process.

- Communicates consultation recommendations that facilitate change.

STANDARD 5D: PRESCRIPTIVE AUTHORITY AND TREATMENT

The advanced practice registered nurse in plastic surgery uses prescriptive authority, procedures, referrals, treatments, and therapies in accordance with state and federal laws and regulations.

Measurement Criteria for the Advanced Practice Registered Nurse:

The advanced practice registered nurse in plastic surgery:

- Prescribes evidence-based treatments, therapies, and procedures for the plastic surgery patient after considering the patient's complete healthcare needs.

- Prescribes pharmacologic agents based on current knowledge and information of pharmacology and physiology.

- Prescribes specific pharmacological agents and/or treatments based on clinical indicators, the plastic surgery patient's status and needs, and the results of diagnostic and laboratory tests.

- Evaluates therapeutic and potential adverse effects of pharmacological and non-pharmacological treatments.

- Provides plastic surgery patients with information about intended effects and potential adverse effects of proposed prescriptive therapies.

- Provides information to the plastic surgery patient about costs, and alternative treatments and procedures, as appropriate.

STANDARD 6: EVALUATION

The plastic surgery nurse evaluates the patient's progress towards achievement of outcomes.

Measurement Criteria:

The plastic surgery registered nurse:

- Conducts a systematic, ongoing, and criterion-based evaluation of the outcomes for the plastic surgery patient in relation to the structures and processes prescribed by the plan and the indicated timeline.

- Includes the plastic surgery patient, appropriate members of the interdisciplinary healthcare team, and others involved in the care or situation in the evaluative process.

- Evaluates the effectiveness of the planned strategies and interventions in relation to the plastic surgery patient's responses and the attainment of the expected outcomes.

- Documents the results of the evaluation.

- Utilizes ongoing assessment data to revise or resolve the diagnoses, the outcomes, the plan of care, and the implementation as needed.

- Disseminates the results of the evaluation to the plastic surgery patient and others involved in the care or situation, as appropriate, in accordance with state and federal laws and regulations.

Additional Measurement Criteria for the Advanced Practice Registered Nurse:

The advanced practice registered nurse in plastic surgery:

- Evaluates the accuracy of the diagnosis and effectiveness of the interventions in relationship to the plastic surgery patient's attainment of expected outcomes.

- Incorporates advanced knowledge, practice, and research into the evaluation process.

- Synthesizes the results of the evaluation analyses to determine the impact of the plan on the affected plastic surgery patients, families, groups, communities, and institutions.

Continued ▶

- Uses the results of the evaluation analyses to make or recommend process or structural changes, including policy, procedure, or protocol documentation, as appropriate.

Standards of Professional Performance

Standard 7. Quality of Practice

The plastic surgery nurse systematically strengthens the quality and effectiveness of nursing practice.

Measurement Criteria:

The plastic surgery nurse:

- Demonstrates quality by documenting the application of the nursing process in a responsible, accountable, and ethical manner.

- Uses the results of quality improvement activities to initiate change in nursing practice and in the healthcare delivery system.

- Uses creativity and innovation in nursing practice to improve care delivery for the plastic surgery patient.

- Incorporates new knowledge to initiate changes in nursing practice if desired outcomes are not achieved.

- Participates in quality improvement activities as appropriate to the nurse's position, education, and practice environment. Activities may include:

  - Identifying aspects of practice important for quality monitoring.

  - Developing indicators that are utilized to monitor the quality and effectiveness of plastic surgery nursing professional practice.

  - Collecting data to monitor quality and effectiveness of plastic surgery nursing practice.

  - Analyzing quality improvement data to recognize opportunities to improve plastic surgery nursing practice.

  - Formulating recommendations to improve plastic surgery nursing care or plastic surgery patient outcomes.

  - Implementing activities to strengthen the quality of nursing practice for the plastic surgery patient.

  - Developing, implementing, and evaluating policies, procedures, and practice guidelines to improve the quality of practice.

  - Participating on multidisciplinary teams to evaluate clinical practice or health services.

Continued ▶

- Taking part in efforts to decrease or minimize costs and redundancy.
- Analyzing factors related to safety and satisfaction, and cost–benefit options associated with quality and effectiveness.
- Analyzing organizational systems for barriers.
- Implementing processes to decrease or remove barriers within organizational systems.

Additional Measurement Criteria for the Advanced Practice Registered Nurse:

The advanced practice registered nurse in plastic surgery:

- Obtains and maintains professional certification in plastic surgery nursing.
- Designs quality improvement initiatives.
- Implements initiatives to evaluate the need for change.
- Evaluates the plastic surgery practice environment and the quality of nursing care using existing evidence, and identifies opportunities for the generation and use of research.

STANDARD 8. EDUCATION

The plastic surgery nurse attains knowledge and competency that reflects current plastic surgery nursing practice.

Measurement Criteria:

The plastic surgery nurse:

- Participates in ongoing educational activities related to practice knowledge and professional issues.

- Demonstrates a commitment to lifelong learning through self-reflection and inquiry to identify learning needs.

- Seeks experiences that reflect current plastic surgery practice in order to develop, maintain, or refine clinical competence or role performance in plastic surgery.

- Acquires knowledge and skills appropriate to the plastic surgery setting, role, or situation by participating in educational programs and activities, conferences, workshops, and interdisciplinary professional meetings.

- Documents and maintains professional records that provide evidence of educational activities, competencies, and lifelong learning.

- Actively and regularly seeks formal and independent learning experiences and opportunities that will advance the nurse's knowledge in plastic surgery, and that meet established goals for professional development.

Additional Measurement Criteria for the Advanced Practice Registered Nurse:

The advanced practice registered nurse in plastic surgery:

- Utilizes current healthcare research findings, scientific findings, and other evidence to expand clinical knowledge, enhance role performance, and increase knowledge of professional issues.

STANDARD 9. PROFESSIONAL PRACTICE EVALUATION

The plastic surgery nurse evaluates one's own nursing practice in relation to professional practice standards and guidelines, relevant statutes, rules, and regulations.

Measurement Criteria:

The plastic surgery nurse's practice reflects the application of knowledge of current practice standards, guidelines, statutes, rules, and regulations.

The plastic surgery nurse:

- Provides age-appropriate care in a culturally and ethnically sensitive manner.

- Engages in a personal performance evaluation on a regular basis, identifying areas of strengths as well as areas in which professional practice development would be beneficial.

- Participates in and seeks informal feedback regarding their own nursing practice and role performance from plastic surgery patients, peers, professional colleagues, and others.

- Participates in systematic peer review as appropriate.

- Takes action to achieve the professional development goals recognized during ongoing and formal performance evaluations.

- Provides rationales for practice beliefs, decisions, and actions as part of the informal and formal evaluation process.

Additional Measurement Criteria for the Advanced Practice Registered Nurse:

The advanced practice registered nurse in plastic surgery:

- Engages in a formal process seeking feedback regarding their own practice from patients, peers, professional colleagues, and others.

Standard 10. Collegiality

The plastic surgery nurse interacts with and contributes to the professional development of peers, colleagues, and other healthcare providers.

Measurement Criteria:

The plastic surgery nurse:

- Shares knowledge, expertise, clinical observations, and skills with peers, colleagues, and other healthcare team members as evidenced by such activities as plastic surgery patient care conferences or presentations at formal or informal meetings.

- Provides peers with constructive feedback regarding their practice and/or role performance.

- Interacts with peers and colleagues to enhance one's own professional nursing practice and/or role performance.

- Contributes to and maintains a supportive and healthy work environment that fosters compassionate and caring relationships with peers and colleagues.

- Contributes to the learning experiences and education of healthcare providers, students, and others through role modeling, acting as a resource, mentoring, or serving as a preceptor or instructor in the plastic surgery clinical setting.

- Differentiates the scope and function of each member of the interdisciplinary healthcare team caring for the plastic surgery patient.

- Contributes to a supportive and healthy plastic surgery work environment.

Additional Measurement Criteria for the Advanced Practice Registered Nurse:

The advanced practice registered nurse in plastic surgery:

- Demonstrates expert practice to interdisciplinary team members and healthcare consumers.

- Mentors and serves as a role model, preceptor, and facilitator of learning in generalist plastic surgery nursing care, in advanced practice plastic surgery nursing, and to other registered nurses and colleagues as appropriate.

Continued ▶

Standards of Professional Performance

- Participates with interdisciplinary teams who contribute to role development and advanced nursing practice and health care.
- Serves as a liaison to institutional, local, state, and national legislative bodies in order to facilitate communication of issues regarding advanced practice in the plastic surgery arena.

STANDARD 11. COLLABORATION

The plastic surgery nurse collaborates with the plastic surgery patient, family, and others in the conduct of nursing practice.

Measurement Criteria:

The plastic surgery nurse:

- Communicates with the plastic surgery patient, family, members of the interdisciplinary healthcare team, and other healthcare providers regarding patient care and the nurse's role in providing that care.

- Collaborates in creating a documented plan focused on outcomes and decisions related to care and delivery of services for the plastic surgery patient, and indicating communication with the plastic surgery patient, family, and appropriate others.

- Coordinates the implementation of care provided for the plastic surgery patient and family by the interdisciplinary healthcare team.

- Partners with others to effect change and generate positive outcomes through knowledge of the plastic surgery patient or situation.

- Documents referrals, including provisions, for continuity of care.

Additional Measurement Criteria for the Advanced Practice Registered Nurse:

The advanced practice registered nurse in plastic surgery:

- Partners with other disciplines to enhance plastic surgery patient care through interdisciplinary activities, such as education, consultation, management, technological development, or research opportunities.

- Contributes to optimizing advanced practice nursing care for the plastic surgery patient in the areas of health education, health promotion, health restoration, and health maintenance.

- Promotes and facilitates an interdisciplinary healthcare process with other members of the healthcare team.

Continued ▶

- Participates in establishing plastic surgery nursing clinical practice guidelines, clinical pathways, and practice protocols.
- Documents the plastic surgery patient's plan of care communications, rationales for plan of care changes, and collaborative discussions to improve his or her care.

STANDARD 12. ETHICS

The plastic surgery nurse integrates ethical provisions in all areas of practice.

Measurement Criteria:

The plastic surgery nurse:

- Utilizes *Code of Ethics for Nurses with Interpretive Statements* (ANA 2001) to guide practice.

- Provides care for the plastic surgery patient in a manner that ensures that the plastic surgery patient's autonomy, dignity, and rights are preserved.

- Maintains plastic surgery patient privacy and confidentiality within legal and regulatory parameters.

- Acts as a patient advocate and liaison, assisting plastic surgery patients in developing skills for self-advocacy.

- Maintains a therapeutic and professional patient–nurse relationship with appropriate professional role boundaries.

- Demonstrates a commitment to practicing self-care, managing stress, and connecting with self and others.

- Recognizes one's own values and beliefs when assisting in the formulation of ethical decisions.

- Contributes to resolving the ethical problems or dilemmas of the plastic surgery patient, colleagues, or systems as evidenced in such activities as participating on ethics committees, and seeking available resources to help formulate ethical decisions.

- Reports abuse of the plastic surgery patient's rights, or illegal, incompetent, or impaired practices.

Additional Measurement Criteria for the Advanced Practice Registered Nurse:

The advanced practice registered nurse in plastic surgery:

- Informs the plastic surgery patient of the risks, benefits, and outcomes of healthcare regimens.

- Participates in interdisciplinary teams that address ethical risks, benefits, and outcomes for the plastic surgery patient.

STANDARD 13. RESEARCH

The plastic surgery nurse integrates research findings into practice.

Measurement Criteria:

The plastic surgery nurse:

- Utilizes the best available evidence, including research findings, to guide practice decisions for the plastic surgery patient.

- Actively participates in research activities at various levels as appropriate to the nurse's level of education and position. Activities may include:

  - Identifying clinical problems specific to nursing research such as patient care and nursing practice.

  - Participating in data collection such as surveys, pilot projects, and formal studies.

  - Participating in a formal committee or program.

  - Sharing research activities and/or findings with peers and others.

  - Conducting research.

  - Critically analyzing and interpreting research findings for application to plastic surgery practice.

  - Utilizing research findings to develop or initiate change in policies, procedures, and standards of practice in plastic surgery patient care.

  - Incorporating research as a basis for learning.

Additional Measurement Criteria for the Advanced Practice Registered Nurse:

The advanced practice registered nurse in plastic surgery:

- Contributes to plastic surgery nursing knowledge by conducting or synthesizing research that discovers, examines, and evaluates knowledge, theories, criteria, and creative approaches to improve healthcare practice for the plastic surgery patient.

- Formally disseminates research findings through activities such as presentations, publications, consultation, and journal clubs.

STANDARD 14. RESOURCE UTILIZATION

The plastic surgery nurse considers factors related to safety, effectiveness, cost, and impact on practice in the planning and delivery of nursing services for the plastic surgery patient.

Measurement Criteria:

The plastic surgery nurse:

- Evaluates factors related to safety, effectiveness, availability, cost and benefits, efficiencies, and impact on practice when choosing among plastic surgery practice options that would result in the same expected outcome.

- Helps the plastic surgery patient and family in identifying and obtaining appropriate and available services to address health-related needs.

- Assigns or delegates tasks, based on the needs and condition of the plastic surgery patient and family, potential for harm, stability of the patient's condition, complexity of the task, and predictability of the outcome.

- Assists the plastic surgery patient and family in becoming informed consumers about the options, costs, risks, and benefits of treatment and care.

Additional Measurement Criteria for the Advanced Practice Registered Nurse:

The advanced practice registered nurse in plastic surgery:

- Utilizes organizational and community resources to formulate multidisciplinary or interdisciplinary plans of care for the plastic surgery patient.

- Develops creative solutions for problems in plastic surgery patient care that address effective resource utilization and maintenance of quality.

- Develops evaluation strategies to demonstrate cost effectiveness, cost benefit, and efficiency factors associated with nursing practice for the plastic surgery patient.

STANDARD 15. LEADERSHIP

The plastic surgery nurse provides leadership in the professional practice setting and the profession.

Measurement Criteria:

The plastic surgery nurse:

- Engages in teamwork as a team player and a team builder.

- Works to create and maintain healthy work environments in local, regional, national, or international communities.

- Displays the ability to define a clear vision, the associated goals, and a plan to implement and measure progress.

- Demonstrates a commitment to continuous, lifelong learning for self and others.

- Teaches others to succeed by mentoring and other strategies.

- Exhibits creativity and flexibility through times of change.

- Demonstrates energy, excitement, and a passion for quality work.

- Willingly accepts mistakes by self and others, thereby creating a culture in which risk-taking is not only safe, but expected.

- Encourages loyalty by valuing people as the most precious asset in an organization.

- Directs the coordination of care across settings and among caregivers, including supervision of licensed and unlicensed personnel in any assigned or delegated tasks as appropriate.

- Serves in important roles in the work setting by participating on committees, councils, and administrative teams.

- Promotes advancement of the profession through participation in professional organizations, such as the American Society of Plastic Surgical Nurses.

Additional Measurement Criteria for the Advanced Practice Registered Nurse:

The advanced practice registered nurse:

- Works to influence decision-making bodies to improve care for the plastic surgery patient.

- Provides direction to enhance the effectiveness of the healthcare team.

- Initiates and revises protocols or guidelines to reflect evidence-based practice, to reflect accepted changes in care management for the plastic surgery patient, or to address emerging problems.

- Promotes communication of information and advancement of the profession through writing, publishing, and presentations for professional or lay audiences.

- Designs innovations to effect change in practice and improve health outcomes.

GLOSSARY

Criteria. Relevant, measurable indicators of the standards of clinical nursing practice.

Healthcare team. A set of individuals with special expertise who provide healthcare services or assistance to patients. They may include nurses, physicians, psychologists, social workers, nutritionists/dieticians, and various therapists. Healthcare providers also may include service organizations and vendors. A team is comprised of a number of persons associated together in work or activity.

Holism (holistic). A view of everything in terms of patterns and processes that combine to form a whole, instead of seeing things as fragments, pieces, or parts. Holistic nursing embraces nursing practice, which has healing the whole person as its goal. Holism involves understanding the individual as an integrated whole interacting with and being acted upon by both internal and external environments.

Interdisciplinary. Reliant on the overlapping skills and knowledge of each team member and discipline, resulting in synergistic effects where outcomes are enhanced and more comprehensive than the simple aggregation of any team member's individual efforts.

Multidisciplinary. Relating to, or using a combination of, several disciplines for a common purpose. A multidisciplinary team is a unit composed of individuals with varied and specialized expertise who coordinate their activities to provide services to patients with an actual or potential diagnosis. The team engages in collaborative endeavors using the combined skills and expertise of team members. The patent is a member of the team whenever possible and appropriate.

Role. A function. The characteristic and expected social behavior of an individual in relationship to a group.

Standard. An authoritative statement enunciated and promulgated by the profession, by which the quality of practice, service, or education can be judged.

REFERENCES

American Board of Medical Specialties. 2000. *Member Boards and Associate Members.* http://www.abms.org/member.asp (accessed February 16, 2004).

American Board of Plastic Surgery. 2003. *About ABPS.* http://www.abplsurg.org/about_abps.html#Description%20of%20Plastic%20Surgery (accessed February 20, 2004).

American Nurses Association. 1995. Committee on Nursing Practices and Guidelines. *Manual to develop guidelines.* Washington, DC: American Nurses Association.

———. 2000. *Scope and standards of practice for nursing professional development.* Washington, DC: nursebooks.org.

———. 2001. *Code of ethics for nurses with interpretive statements.* Washington, DC: ANA.

———. 2003. *Nursing's social policy statement,* 2nd edition. Washington, DC: ANA.

———. 2004. *Nursing: Scope and standards of practice.* Washington, DC: ANA.

American Society of Plastic and Reconstructive Surgical Nurses. 2002. *About ASPSN.* http://www.aspsn.org/ABOUT/objectives.html (accessed March 16, 2004).

American Society of Plastic Surgeons. 2004. *Procedural statistics trends 1992–2003.* http://www.plasticsurgery.org/public_education/Statistical-Trends.cfm (accessed March 16, 2004).

BIBLIOGRAPHY

American Society of Plastic and Reconstructive Surgical Nurses. 1987. *Standards for plastic surgical nurses.* Pitman, NJ: ASPRSN.

———. 1996. *Standards for plastic surgical nurses,* 2nd edition. Pitman, NJ: ASPRSN.

———. 1996. *Core curriculum for plastic and reconstructive surgical nursing,* 2nd edition. Pitman, NJ: American Society of Plastic Surgical Nurses.

Association of periOperative Registered Nurses. 2001. *Standards, recommended practices and guidelines.* Denver, CO: AORN.

Brunner, L., and Suddarth, D. 2000. *Textbook of medical surgical nursing.* Philadelphia: Lippincott.

Carpenito, L. 2004. *Nursing diagnosis: Application to clinical practice.* Philadelphia: Lippincott.

Dermatology Nurses Association. 2002. *Dermatology nursing scope of practice and dermatology nursing standards of clinical practice.* Pitman, NJ: DNA.

Goodman, T., ed. 1988. *Core curriculum for plastic and reconstructive surgical nursing.* Pitman, NJ: American Society of Plastic Surgical Nurses.

INDEX

A

Accreditation Association for Ambulatory Health Care (AAAHC), 11, 13
Advanced practice plastic surgery nursing
  assessment, 19–20
  collaboration, 39–40
  collegiality, 37–38
  consultation, 29
  coordination of care, 27
  defined, 7
  diagnosis, 21
  education, 35
  ethics, 41
  evaluation, 31–32
  health teaching and health promotion, 28
  implementation, 26
  leadership, 44–45
  outcomes identification, 22–23
  planning, 24–25
  prescriptive authority and treatment, 30
  professional practice evaluation, 36
  quality of practice, 33–34
  research, 42
  resource utilization, 43
  roles, 7–8
  See also Generalist plastic surgery nursing; Plastic surgery nursing
Advertising, 16
  See also Media coverage
Advocacy for patients and families, 1
  ethics and, 15–17, 41
Aesthetic plastic surgery, 2, 3, 9, 12
  ethics and, 16, 17
  media coverage, 1, 6
  population, 15
  See also Plastic surgery; Reconstructive plastic surgery
Age-appropriate care. *See* Cultural competence

Aging population, 16
American Association for Accreditation of Ambulatory Surgery Facilities (AAAASF), 11–12, 13
American Board of Medical Specialties, 1
American Board of Plastic Surgery (ABPS), 1, 16
American Nurses Association (ANA), 2
  Code of Ethics with Interpretive Statements, 15, 41
  Nursing's Social Policy Statement, 5
American Society of Plastic and Reconstructive Surgical Nurses (ASPRSN), 3, 4
American Society of Plastic Surgeons (ASPS), 2, 3, 12, 16
American Society of Plastic Surgical Nurses (ASPSN), 3, 4, 5, 44
Americans with Disabilities Act, 12, 13
Analysis. *See* Critical thinking, analysis, and synthesis
Assessment, 5, 8, 9, 11, 12, 13, 14, 15
  diagnosis and, 21
  evaluation and, 31
  planning and, 24
  standard of practice, 19–20
Association of periOperative Registered Nurses (AORN), 2

B

Body of knowledge of plastic surgery nursing, 1, 7, 8, 9, 11
  assessment and, 20
  collaboration and, 7, 39
  development of, 3, 5, 7
  education and, 9, 35
  evaluation and, 31
  planning and, 24
  prescriptive authority and treatment, 30
  quality of practice and, 33
  requirements, 6, 14, 15
  research and, 9, 42

Ethics (*continued*)
  quality of practice and, 33
  standard of professional
    performance, 41
  See also Code of Ethics for Nurses
    with Interpretive Statements;
    Laws, statutes, and regulations
Evaluation, 5, 9, 10, 15
  in practice settings, 11, 13
  resource utilization and, 43
  standard of practice, 31–32
Evidence-based practice, 5, 9
  assessment and, 19
  consultation and, 29
  education and, 35
  implementation and, 26
  leadership and, 45
  outcomes identification and, 22
  planning and, 24
  prescriptive authority and
    treatment, 30
  quality of practice and, 34
  See also Body of knowledge; Research

F
Family, 10, 14
  assessment and, 19
  collaboration and, 39
  coordination of care and, 27
  diagnosis and, 21
  evaluation and, 31
  health teaching and health
    promotion, 28
  outcomes identification and, 22
  planning and, 24
  resource utilization and, 43
  See also Education of patients and
    families; Patient
Financial issues. *See* Cost control

G
Generalist plastic surgery nursing
  assessment, 19
  collaboration, 39
  collegiality, 37
  coordination of care, 27

diagnosis, 21
education, 35
ethics, 41
evaluation, 31
health teaching and health
  promotion, 28
implementation, 26
leadership, 44
outcomes identification, 22
planning, 24
professional practice evaluation, 36
quality of practice, 33–34
research, 42
resource utilization, 43
roles, 7
See also Advanced plastic surgery
  nursing; Plastic surgery nursing
Guidelines, 5, 8, 9
  collaboration and, 39
  outcomes identification and, 23

H
Health Insurance Portability and
  Accountability Act (HIPAA), 11, 19
Health teaching and health promotion,
  2, 5, 7, 8, 14
  collaboration and, 39
  planning and, 24
  in practice settings, 13, 15
  standard of practice, 28
  resource utilization and, 43
Healthcare policy, 10
  evaluation and, 32
  quality of practice and, 33
  research and, 42
Healthcare providers, 2, 8, 10, 13
  assessment and, 19
  collaboration and, 39
  collegiality and, 37
  diagnosis and, 21
  leadership and, 44
  outcomes identification and, 22
  planning and, 24
  quality of practice and,
  See also Collaboration;
    Interdisciplinary health car

Nursing care standards. *See* Standards of care

Nursing process, 1, 2, 5, 11
    collaboration and, 39
    quality of practice and, 33
    See also Standards of Practice

Nursing standards. *See* Standards of practice; Standards of professional performance

O

Occupational Safety and Health Administration (OSHA), 12

Outcomes identification, 5, 11
    standard of practice, 22–23
    See also Outcomes

Outcomes, 2, 5, 8, 9, 10
    collaboration and, 39
    diagnosis and, 21
    ethics and, 41
    evaluation and, 31
    implementation and, 26
    planning and, 24
    quality of practice and, 33
    resource utilization and, 43
    See also Evaluation; Outcomes identification

P

Parents. *See* Family

Patient
    assessment and, 19
    collaboration and, 39
    consultation and, 29
    coordination of care and, 27
    diagnosis and, 21
    ethics and, 41
    evaluation and, 31
    health teaching and promotion, 28
    outcomes identification and, 22
    planning and, 24
    prescriptive authority and treatment, 30
    professional practice evaluation and, 36
    resource utilization and, 43
    rights, 15–16

    See also Education of patients and families; Family

Patient population, 14–15, 16

Pharmacologic agents. *See* Prescriptive authority

Planning, 2, 5, 9, 14
    collaboration and, 39, 40
    consultation and, 29
    coordination of care and, 27
    diagnosis and, 21
    evaluation and, 31
    implementation and, 26
    leadership and, 44
    outcomes identification and, 22
    in practice settings, 10, 11, 12, 13
    standard of practice, 24–25

Plastic surgery
    demand, 1, 2, 16
    media coverage, 1–2, 5
    patient population, 14–15, 16
    psychological effects, 2, 5, 9, 14, 24
    risks, 2, 12, 16
    stages, 2, 9, 11, 12, 13
    See also Aesthetic plastic surgery; Reconstructive plastic surgery

Plastic surgery nurse educator, 8–9
    See also Education of plastic surgery nurses

Plastic surgery nursing
    advanced practice, 7–8
    body of knowledge, 1, 2, 3, 5, 6, 7, 8, 9, 11, 14, 15
    certification, 1, 4, 6, 8, 11, 12, 16
    characteristics, 1–2
    defined, 1
    generalist practice, 7
    history, 2–5
    minimum requirements, 6
    research, 3, 5, 7, 8, 9–10
    roles, 5–9
    scope of practice, 1–17
    standards of practice, *vii–viii*, 19–32
    standards of professional performance, *ix*, 33–45
    trends, 2, 3–4, 7, 12, 16
    See also Advanced practice plastic

surgery nursing; Generalist
plastic surgery nursing
Plastic surgery nursing advanced level.
See Advanced practice plastic
surgery nursing
Plastic Surgical Nursing Certification
Board (PSNCB), 4, 6
Plastic Surgical Nursing Journal, 4
Policy. See Healthcare policy
Practice environment, 9, 10–11, 15
collegiality and, 37
coordination of care and, 27
leadership and, 44
outcomes identification and, 22
quality of practice and, 33
Practice settings, 3, 5, 15, 16
hospital, 11
nursing roles, 8, 9
office-based surgery center, 12–13
outpatient/ambulatory surgery
center, 11–12
private practice, 13–14
Preceptors. See Mentoring
Prescriptive authority and treatment, 8
standard of practice, 30
Privacy. See Confidentiality
Process. See Nursing process
Professional development,
education and, 35
professional practice evaluation
and, 36
See also Education; Leadership
Professional organizations,
Professional performance. See
Standards of professional
performance
Professional practice evaluation
collegiality and, 37
health teaching and health
promotion, 28
standard of professional
performance, 36

Q
Quality of life, 10, 28
Quality of practice, 5, 9, 10, 13, 15

outcomes identification and, 22
standard of professional
performance, 33–34

R
Recipient of care. See Patient
Reconstructive plastic surgery, 1, 2, 3, 9, 12
ethics and, 17
population, 14–15
See also Aesthetic plastic surgery;
Plastic surgery
Referrals. See Collaboration;
Coordination of care
Regulatory issues. See Laws, statutes,
and regulations
Reimbursement, 8, 17
Research, 3, 4, 5, 9–10
collaboration and, 39
defined, 9
education and, 35
evaluation and, 31
implementation and, 26
nursing roles, 7, 8, 9–10
planning and, 24
quality of practice and, 34
standard of professional
performance, 42
See also Evidence-based practice
Resource utilization
ethics and, 41
health teaching and health
promotion, 28
implementation and, 26
outcomes identification and, 22
standard of professional
performance, 43
Risk assessment, 2, 12, 16
ethics and, 41
health teaching and health
promotion, 28
leadership and, 44
outcomes identification and, 22
prescriptive authority and
treatment, 30
resource utilization and, 43
Role (defined), 47

ANA Nursing Standards Package

The set—totaling over 1,200 pages—contains the newly revised keystone publication of the set, *Nursing: Scope and Standards of Practice*, plus one each of the current volume for the 19 nursing specialty areas listed below. Each volume delineates and discusses the scope, status, and prospects of that specialized practice along with its generalist competencies, any advanced practice competencies, and the evidence-based standards with measurement criteria for practice and professional performance. **Pub #PKG**   *List $295 / Member $260*

The ANA Nursing Standards Package contains:

Nursing: Scope and Standards of Practice, 2004/168 pp. (*NEW EDITION*)
Includes the standards for clinical, non-clinical, and advanced practice, and the 1973,1981,1991,1996,and 1998 editions.
#04SSNP   **List $19.95 / Member $16.95**

... plus 19 additional scope and standards of specialty practice.* **All affordably priced at List $16.95/Member $13.45:**

The latest additions to the set...

Nurse Administrators, 2004 (*NEW EDITION*)	#03SSNA	
Addictions Nursing, 2004 (*NEW EDITION*)	#04SSAN	
Intellectual & Dvlptl Disabilities Nursing (*NEW*)	#04SSID	
Pain Management Nursing, 2005 (*1st EDITION*)	#05SSPM	
Plastic Surgery Nursing, 2005 (*1st EDITION*)	#05SSPS	
Neonatal Nursing, 2004 (*1st EDITION*)	#04SSNN	
Vascular Nursing, 2004 (*1st EDITION*)	#04SSVN	

... have joined these titles:

Diabetes Nursing (2nd EDITION), 2003	#DNP23
Gerontological Nursing, (2nd EDITION), 2001	#GNP21
Home Health Nursing, 1999	#9905HH
Neuroscience Nursing, 2002	#NNS22
Nursing Informatics, 2001	#NIP21
Nursing Professional Development, 2000	#NPD20
Palliative & Hospice Nursing, 2002	#HPN22

Parish Nursing, 1998	#9806ST
Pediatric Nursing, 2003 (*NEW EDITION*)	#PNP23
Pediatric Oncology Nursing, 2000	#PONP20
Psychiatric–Mental Health Nursing, 2000	#PMH20
Public Health Nursing, 1999	#9910PH

Coming summer 2005:
School Nursing: Scope & Standards of Practice (*NEW EDITION*)

ANA Standards Standing Order Plan
Great plan for university, hospital, and medical center libraries! Get the newest Standards as soon as they are published. We'll send the book along with an invoice. Plus, you'll save 10% off list price.
(*ANA members receive an additional 20% savings.*)
For details, or to enroll, call (800) 637-0323.

(* Titles may be ordered separately. New and revised titles are being added continually.)

ORDER FORM

Title	Price	Qty	Total
ANA Nursing Standards Package #PKG			
	Shipping & Handling		
	TOTAL		

Shipping and Handling		
	U.S.	Outside U.S.
Up to $25	$4	$8
$25.01–$50	$6	$12
$50.01–$100	$8	$16
$100.01–$200	$14	$24
$200.01–$300	$12	$32
$300.01 +	7% of total	15% of total

Payment: (payment in U.S. dollars required)
[ ] Check enclosed (made payable to *American Nurses Association*)
Charge my [ ] VISA   [ ] MasterCard

Card # _____ Exp Date _____

Signature _____

Phone # _____ CMA# _____ **

***Your CMA I.D. number must be provided to receive member discount.**.

20% discount off list price on orders of 20+ copies of the same title.

Shipping: 7 to10 business days for domestic deliveries. 7 to 30 business days for international deliveries. Items cannot be delivered to a P.O. box.
All orders must include shipping and handling charges.

Ship to:
Name _____

Organization _____

Address _____

City/State/Zip _____

Phone # _____ Fax # _____

HOW TO ORDER
📖 **Online:** WWW.NURSESBOOKS.ORG 📖 **Phone**: 800/637-0323 📖 **Fax:** 770/280-4141
📖 **Mail:** nursesbooks.org, P.O. Box 931895, Atlanta, GA 31193-1895

DATE DUE
